SIX HEALING OILS

YOU CAN'T LIVE WITHOUT AND MORE!

Super Dirt Cheap Healers You Just Have To Know About Today!

...boost the immune system, even though it is not completely understood how it works!

Brought dramatic relief to inflammation and stiff joints caused by rheumatoid arthritis!

Seriously ill cancer patients were treated... 90 days, tumors gradually receded!

The antiseptic powers... are GIGANTIC...!

... remove toxins like mercury from the body!

far less heart disease than Americans, ... they drink, smoke, consumed more saturated fat...!

is a POTENT CLEANSER - DETOXIFIER!

...period of approximately 90 days, tumors gradually receded!

TOP SECRET! Includes 01 More SUPER HEALER You Just Have To Know About Today!!

100% Satisfaction Guarantee

JOSEPH A. LAYDON JR.

"Six Healing Oils You Can't Live Without And More!"

UPDATED: 312003C August 2023 (Thursday)

Published By Joseph A. Laydon Jr.

Website: https://www.survivalexpertblog.com

E-Mail: wwwsurvivalexpert@yahoo.com

MOST IMPORTANT NOTE: The individual *"Six Healing Oils You Can't Live Without And More!"* is a compilation from my already published Anytime Anywhere Survival Newsletters (AASN) at https://www.survivalexpertblog.com

Published By: Joseph A. Laydon Jr.

Website: https://www.survivalexpertblog.com

E-Mail: wwwsurvivalexpert@yahoo.com

Copyright & Disclaimer

IRISAP DISCLAIMER STATEMENT

The author of *"Six Healing Oils You Can't Live Without And More!"* and owner of Intensive Research Information Services And Product(s) (IRISAP) is exercising his right under the First Amendment to self-publish and co-author this informational product to better educate the public with respect to being more self-reliant Anytime Anywhere. The author is publishing this information based upon his *"intensive research"* and his experiences. Author is demonstrating through this Survival Book how to become self-reliant in survival situations.

This Survival Book is designed to help the reader become more aware of the unique applications of Alternative Therapies like Oils.

The information within this Survival Book is for educational purposes only. Professional advice from *"qualified medical professionals "* is ALWAYS and HIGHLY recommended. Advice is neither implied nor intended. IRISAP and authors\writers of resource materials are not responsible for the purchaser's and third party activities and is in no way responsible for sickness or death or successes.

THE PURCHASER OF THIS SPECIAL REPORT IS SOLELY RESPONSIBLE FOR THIRD PARTY DISCLOSURE AND RESPONSIBLE FOR THEIR ACTIONS AND ANY PRIVATE OR PROFESSIONAL ACTIONS TAKEN FROM THIS INFORMATIONAL PRODUCT. This Special Report is Copyrighted and VIOLATORS WILL BE PROSECUTED!

If the consumer DISAGREES with ANY portion of this DISCLAIMER STATEMENT, the consumer MUST immediately (upon receipt) return this entire informational product for a full refund.

Table Of Contents

Contents

Dedication!

This book - *"Six Healing Oils You Can't Live Without And More!"* is dedicated to all the past, present and future sickly and dead patients who put their total trust in conventional medicine of drugs and surgery.

There are better alternatives to the multitudes of sickly therapies of drugs used in conventional medicine.

There are more than 60 Alternative Therapies. 60 Alternative Therapies that are worthy of your attention. The 600+-page Gettysburg Program found at **www.survivalexpertblog.com/52-survival-books** is where the Gettysburg Program and other data can be found concerning Alternative Therapies used throughout the world and throughout history.

This Book - *"Six Healing Oils You Can't Live Without And More!"* barely, barely, barely touches all those 60+ Alternative Therapies. I highly encourage you to see all my Books for much more Self-Reliance Data. See More Kindle Books and Paperback Book at the end of this book.

And don't forget to see Survival Expert at **www.survivalexpertblog.com**

Introduction

Welcome to *Six Healing Oils You Can't Live Without And More!*"

Welcome and thank you for getting ***"Six Healing Oils You Can't Live Without And More!"*** where you'll find real <u>healthy</u> survival information that will compliment any other healthy survival knowledge you may already possess. Learn these "healthy healing oil survival tricks" so you're ready Anytime Anywhere.

Somebody in your family household has to be the Survival Expert – even when it comes to alternative healthcare when conventional medicine has failed. Somebody has to be the Survival Expert, why not you? And here's a good start so you're ready Anytime Anywhere!

IMPORTANT NOTE: ***"Six Healing Oils You Can't Live Without and More!*** is not in alphabetical order. I encourage you to read this Book multiple times so you're ready Anytime Anywhere!

THIS PAGE IS BLANK

"Six Healing Oils You Can't Live Without And More!"

Here are *"Six Healing Oils You Can't Live Without And More"* that are worthy of your attention. OK, let's start with *Healing Benefits Of Shark Liver Oil*.

NOTE: These *"Six Healing Oils You Can't Live Without And More* <u>**are not in alphabetical order**</u> and are direct quotes from several Anytime Anywhere Survival Newsletters from the *2012 Ultra-Advanced Anytime Anywhere Survival Program TOTAL Package (2012 U-AAASPTP)*.

"Italy and Greece have lower heart disease and stroke"

...help protect arteries and blood vessels by significantly lowering bad-type blood cholesterol (LDL)

"...brought dramatic relief to inflammation and stiff joints caused by rheumatoid arthritis."

used for centuries for common colds, flues, minor aches and inflammation *"the consumption of as little as one or two fish dishes per week may be of preventive importance in relation to coronary heart disease."*

"People in the Mediterranean have been noted to develop far less heart disease than Americans"

"Mediterranean groups had lower death rates, longer life expectancies in Greece than in any other European or North American country despite their high tobacco consumption, low exercise level and modest health-care system"

...researchers have successfully blocked both migraine headaches and kidney disease...
"...ameliorating, healing, reversing, preventing: accelerated wound healing, allergies, asthma, atherosclerosis, brain tumors including other cancers, Candida fungus..."

"...successfully blocked both migraine headaches and kidney disease..."

...rates high for keeping blood pressure in a healthy range. Jichi Medical School in Japan have shown that levels of "good" HDL cholesterol were high among Japanese...

"Oregano could turn into the next wonder drug."

I have to tell you about the healing benefits of ____ remarkable healing and health enhancing oils!

Shark Liver Oil

Olive Oil

Omega-3 Fatty Acids

Castor Oil

Flaxseed Oil

Oil Of Oregano

OK, let's get started with *"Healing Benefits Of Shark Liver Oil."*

"Healing Benefits Of Shark Liver Oil!"

Initially a Scandinavian folk medicine, Shark Liver Oil has been used for centuries for common colds, flues, minor aches and inflammation. Shark Liver Oil has now drawn the attention of scientist, doctors and health enthusiast all around the world!

Its early research focused on enhancing the immune system, radiation treatment protection, and reduction in the mortality rate of cancer patients.

Health enthusiast have noted benefits of Shark Liver Oil such as ameliorating, healing, reversing, preventing: accelerated wound healing, allergies, asthma, atherosclerosis, brain tumors including other cancers, Candida fungus, colds, chronic fatigue syndrome, cosmetic decline, flu...

What gives Shark Liver Oil its healing benefits? Shark Liver Oil contains squalene, omega-3 oils (EPA & DHA), alkylglycerols (AKGs), and other substances, but for this IRISAP Special Report, we'll talk about the special healing ingredients above.

What is squalene?
An element of shark oils, squalene is generally related to Vitamin A. Some shark livers contain as much as 65% squalene by weight.

Used in the cosmetic industry, it is noted to benefit the skin with the use of skin moisturizers.

What are Alkylglycerols (AKGs)?

AKGs support the requirements of the white blood cell (immune system). Oil-based chelating agents, AKGs remove toxins like mercury from the body. Benefits of AKGs are noted to be:

- anti-bacterial
- anti-fungal
- anti-inflammatory (arthritis)
- arterial walls become more elastic
- asthma
- heavy metals are removed via oil-based chelating.
- immune system enhancement
- inhibits blood clots
- lowering LDL cholesterol (bad cholesterol)
- promotes vasodilatation (lowers blood pressure)
- protection from radiation
- psoriasis and other skin problems
- raising HDL cholesterol (good cholesterol)

Can AKGs really support my immune system?

AKGs are noted to boost the immune system, even though it is not completely understood how it works. AKGs are instrumental in production and stimulation of white blood cells in bone marrow. Besides Shark Liver Oil, AKGs are found in saltwater & freshwater fish, cows, and sheep.

Mother's milk has 10-times more AKG's than cow's milk. Your liver, spleen and bone marrow (part of the immune system), have AKGs. However, the most AKGs are found in deep water sharks!

Where can I get these AKGs?
AKGs are just one component of Shark Liver Oil. An authentic Shark Liver Oil product can be acquired from companies listed below at the end of this Special Report.

What about the other ingredient in Shark Liver Oil, Omega-3 oils?
Heart-health experts have found the benefits of eating fish are even greater than previously realized. In 1985 the New England Journal of Medicine found that *"the consumption of as little as one or two fish dishes per week may be of preventive importance in relation to coronary heart disease."* Omega-3 fats in fish benefits the heart by making the blood less prone to the abnormal clotting process that can lead to a heart attack.

Fresh fish rates high for keeping blood pressure in a healthy range. Jichi Medical School in Japan have shown that levels of *"good"* HDL cholesterol were high among Japanese who eat the most fish! Fish may also help those who suffer from arthritis.

According to Dr. Joel Kremer of Albany Medical College in New York, daily supplements of EPA (eicosapentaenoic acid) fish oil brought dramatic relief to inflammation and stiff joints caused by rheumatoid arthritis.

According to researchers at the University of Cincinnati, Ohio, researchers have successfully blocked both migraine headaches and kidney disease with Omega-3 fish oils. Migraines generally eased up in about 60 percent of those who took fish oil capsules for six weeks. The number of migraine attacks dropped from 02 per week to 02 every 02 weeks and they were less severe!

Those patients diagnosed early of kidney disease, showed a retardation of kidney deterioration by switching from animal fat to Omega-3 fish oils. According to Dr. Uno Barcelli, assistant professor of medicine at the University of Cincinnati, *"It seems fish oil must be used relatively early in the disease process."* Fish oil therapy had no effect on patients with advanced kidney disease.

Remember, to acquire an authentic Shark Liver Oil supplement, please do your own research and ask folks at your local healthfood store.

"Natural Healing Benefits of Olive Oil!"

Olive oil varies in quality. The term *"virgin"* is loosely applied. Originally it meant that the oil was from the first pressing of the fruit, as opposed to the second or third pressing. Olive oil when unrefined has a greenish tinge and a pungent flavor. It is preferred to refined oils because the health qualities are intact.

Olive oil may be one of the best choices when cooking with oils. Olive oil IS NOT saturated fat but is a monounsaturated fatty acid, which is stable at high temperatures and less prone to oxidation than other vegetable oils. Extra Virgin Oil is probably your best choice of all the other oils.

People in the Mediterranean have been noted to develop far less heart disease than Americans, even though they drink, smoke and even consumed as much or more saturated fat than Americans! What are they doing different? Their diet consists of an oil they use on their vegetables, grain-rich dishes and meats. They even dip their bread in it! It's olive oil!

Yes, olive oil. One added bonus of monounsaturated fats, they maintain HDL (high density lipoprotein) that helps prevent heart disease. Olive, peanut and canola oils are noted to be highest in monounsaturated fats.

Insure you read the Nutrition Facts label on any cooking oil. Look for the word *"monounsaturated."* Look for the least amount of saturated fats and the most monounsaturated fats.

WARNING: INSURE you use *"cold pressed"* olive oil - Extra Virgin Olive Oil! Use all cooking oils sparingly!

Why are people who live by the Mediterranean Diet, healthier than Americans despite their high tobacco consumption, low exercise level and modest health-care system?

The Mediterranean Diet is a diet low in meat, but high in cereal, fruit, grain, legumes, monounsaturated fats-nuts and vegetables. Recent French Study found that the Mediterranean Diet after a heart attack was 70 percent more life-saving than the Standard American Diet (low-fat diet-less than 30 percent fat calories). Some Harvard Researchers favor the Mediterranean Diet over the Standard American Diet.

A research effort called the Seven Countries Study, examined 12,763 men ages 40 through 59 in the Netherlands, Finland, Italy, Greece, Croatia and Serbia, Japan and the United States. Ten years after their initial screening, the study reported several important results:

- Mediterranean groups had lower death rates from all causes than the northern European and American groups.

- Lower mortality from coronary heart disease in Mediterranean countries.

- Men at the peak of their lives (45 years) have longer life expectancies in Greece than in any other European or North American country despite their high tobacco consumption, low exercise level and modest health-care system.

The Mediterranean Diet is based on traditional eating patterns evolving over centuries in Greece, Italy, North Africa, Southern France, Spain and several Middle Eastern nations. All share a general pattern of cooking and ingredients. The diet is rich in fruits, vegetables, legumes and grains.

The principal fat is olive oil! Lean red meat is eaten only a few times a month and in small portions. Eating foods from animal sources - namely dairy products, fish and poultry is low to moderate. Wine is drunk with meals. Plenty of crusty country-style bread is enjoyed with each meal.

The major fat used in the Mediterranean Diet is olive oil! Olive oil is primarily a monounsaturated fat, which is noted to lower harmful low-density lipoprotein (LDL) blood cholesterol and may increase good high-density lipoprotein (HDL) blood cholesterol.

Olive oil isn't the only key to a healthy diet.
Here are some Mediterranean eating tips:

- Switch to olive oil (extra virgin).

- Avoid butter and margarine. There is nothing wrong with putting olive oil on toast or whole grain bread.

- Cut meat consumption. If you do eat meat, insure it's lean. Try small portions of poultry or fish with plenty of vegetables.

- INCREASE fruit and vegetable consumption.

- Eat plenty of whole grain bread. The darker the better (ingredients not burnt).

- Eat a salad at the beginning and end of each meal.

- Wine at each dinner meal. It's been noted that a couple glasses of wine each day may protect against coronary heart disease.

"You Gotta Have Your Omega-3 Fattys Acids For Lunch And Dinner!"

Omega-3 Fatty Acids are made up of two components DHA & EPA! DHA which stands for docosahexaenoic acid. EPA stands for eicosapentaenoic acid. These two nutrients found in Omega-3 are noted to protect against heart disease, stroke, depression...

It was once thought that shellfish were hazardous to your cardiovascular system because they elevated blood cholesterol. Well it is just the opposite. Shellfish help protect arteries and blood vessels by significantly lowering bad-type blood cholesterol (LDL).

Shellfish carry high concentrations of Omega-3 fatty acids that help prevent blood clots (thrombi) in blood vessels and are noted to be potentially beneficial to many diseases to include allergies, asthma, cancer, headaches, psoriasis and rheumatoid arthritis!

Heart-health experts have found the benefits of eating fish are even greater than previously realized. In 1985 the New England Journal of Medicine found that *"the consumption of as little as one or two fish dishes per week may be of preventive importance in relation to coronary heart disease."*

Omega-3 fats in fish benefits the heart by making the blood less prone to the abnormal clotting process that can lead to a heart attack.

Fresh fish rates high for keeping blood pressure in a healthy range. Jichi Medical School in Japan have shown that levels of *"good"* HDL cholesterol were high among Japanese who eat the most fish! Fish may also help those who suffer from arthritis.

According to Dr. Joel Kremer of Albany Medical College in New York, daily supplements of EPA (eicosapentaenoic acid) fish oil brought dramatic relief to inflammation and stiff joints caused by rheumatoid arthritis.

Fish is less fattening and more digestible than beef. Fish is high in mineral selenium which has proven to chase away the blues. There are about twenty varieties of fish that can be purchased at your local supermarket. Four ounces of fish furnishes anywhere from 89 calories to 236 calories, with raw haddock having the lowest calorie count of 89 and four ounces of canned herring rates the highest calorie count of 236.

- Salmon is low in saturated fat and high in Omega-3 fatty acids. Salmon provides only 233 calories per 4.5 ounce steak and only 6 grams of fat per 3 ounces.

According to researchers at the University of Cincinnati, Ohio, researchers have successfully blocked both migraine headaches and kidney disease with Omega-3 fish oils. Migraines generally eased up in about 60 percent of those who took fish oil capsules for six weeks. The number of migraine attacks dropped from 02 per week to 02 every 02 weeks and they were less severe!

Those patients diagnosed early of kidney disease, showed a retardation of kidney deterioration by switching from animal fat to Omega-3 fish oils. According to Dr. Uno Barcelli, assistant professor of medicine at the University of Cincinnati, *"It seems fish oil must be used relatively early in the disease process."* Fish oil therapy had no effect on patients with advanced kidney disease.

English Nuts are five times more rich in Omega-3 fatty acids than all other nuts. Very few plant foods have this much Omega-3 fatty acids. English Nuts are also high in antioxidant anticancer allagic acid.

DHA an important essential fatty acid (Omega-3), is a major building block in gray matter of your brain. It also a major building block of the retina of your eye.

According to American Journal of Clinical Nutrition, *"Societies consuming large amounts of fish and Omega-3 fatty acids appear to have lower rates of major depression."*

WARNING: Fast food fish is noted to have 1/10 of Omega-3 fish oil compared to a can of Chinook salmon. Fast food fish is mostly made from whitefish already low in fat and Omega-3's. Too much Omega-3 may block normal blood clotting and lead to excessive bleeding. Researchers have discovered that Omega-3 fish oil capsules can actually aggravate diabetes by producing a steep rise in blood sugar and a drop in insulin secretion.

"Amazing Healing Castor Oil!"

Can you give me some general information about Castor Oil?

Castor Oil is extracted from the castor bean plant and it's been used for thousands of years for just about every malady - sickness you can think of!

Castor Oil packs (more on this later) have been used with amazing results that most medical doctors would say is impossible. It is even taken internally.

Ask your own physician about the healing qualities and successes of Castor Oil. He\she may probably just laugh or discredit you and tell you to stay away from that nonsense! You have the right to investigate any alternative - at least look into it.

Many varieties of sickly and deadly maladies have responded positively to the amazing healing qualities of Castor Oil. Castor Oil is a POTENT CLEANSER - DETOXIFIER! This means it gives your cleansed body the inherent ability to heal itself!

What is Castor Oil composed of?

Castor Oil is mainly composed of ricinoleic acid. Ricinoleic acid is an unsaturated hydroxy fatty acid. A high viscosity oil, some have described it as a nutritious oil.

It's noted to be an excellent emollient and lubricant as well as demonstrating antimicrobial activities. Below is a composition of Castor Oil:

Ricinoleic acid--------------------89.5%
Oleic acid------------------------03.0%
Palmitic acid---------------------01.0%
Stearic acid----------------------01.0%
Dihydroxystearic acid-------------00.7%
Eicosanoic acid-------------------00.3%
Linoleic acid---------------------00.3%
Linolenic acid--------------------00.3%

What is the healing secret to Castor Oil?
First of all, like many natural and extremely safe supplements like herbs, foods (raw fresh fruits & vegetables), miracle waters, other oils..., and 60 remarkable alternative healing therapies & treatments, research needs to be conducted! Research results you may NEVER see! Not in your lifetime.

Why many natural supplements and alternative therapies work - exactly work is unknown! There is a lot of good scientific evidence why many supplements work and why some Alternative Therapies work. But to find the EXACT reason why they any healing takes place needs much more research.

Heck, scientist and researchers are still conducting research on water - plain ol' water! I forget the name of the field of studying water - but that's all these scientists and researchers do - study water! And they'll be doing it as long as there is money to finance the research!

To come up with bonafide reasons why Castor Oil works along with hundreds of other alternative supplements and treatments & therapies - well don't hold your breath.

My best advice is to try to go back to the basics which is to use common sense and do what your doctor advises (as long as it works) and ALWAYS keep an open mind to other Alternatives Therapies that are safe and help your body to heal itself!

What are some healing benefits of Castor Oil?
The following is a partial list of reported healing results using Castor Oil packs. For many of the maladies listed below, a Castor Oil Pack on the abdomen has demonstrated remarkable results. Later you'll see how to make these healing Castor Oil packs.

- abdominal problems
- aching feet
- acne
- appendicitis

- arthritis
- back pain
- bath pruitis (itching)
- beautiful complexion
- cancer
- colitis
- constipation
- corns
- cyst
- ear problems
- edema of the ankles
- esophagus
- flactuance
- gall bladder conditions
- hearing loss
- hematoma (bleeding under the skin)
- hernias
- Hodgkin's Disease
- hyperactivity (tranquilizing effect)*
- inflammations
- liver conditions
- insomnia
- irregular-painful toe nails
- lesion
- liver spots
- migraine headaches
- Multiple Sclerosis
- nausea - vomiting

- pain
- Parkinson's Disease
- Ringworm
- sciatic pain
- severe skin abrasions (sans scars)
- skin abrasions
- skin cancer
- skin rash
- smashed or crushed finger - toe nails
- snoring (Castor Oil pack placed on abdomen)
- sprained ankle
- stretch marks
- vaginitis
- varicose veins
- warts
- Castor Oil pack on the belly.

How do I make Castor Oil Packs?

First of all, INSURE you have the cooperation and support of your doctor when using Castor Oil. Also insure you read additional and revealing information on Castor Oil (see below).

Below is a step-by-step list for making Castor Oil Packs:

a) Gather the following items:
   01) Bath Towel (white)
   02) Castor Oil (see Point of Contact)

03) Clear plastic sheet
04) Electric heating pad
05) Flannel cloth - large (wool)
06) Pan (10 x 14 inches)
06) Safety pins

b) Take your flannel cloth and fold it so that it is 2 to four layers and measures 10 by 14 inches. I'll give you a POC that offers Castor Oil as well as reusable wool flannel (18 X 24-abdominal & 12 X 18-other areas). Place the flannel cloth in the pan.

c) Pour Castor Oil in the pan and completely saturate the entire wool flannel cloth.

d) Remove the flannel and remove excess Castor Oil by wringing it out in the pan - but it must be wet but not dripping wet.

e) Apply the saturated flannel cloth to the abdomen (stimulates the thymus - immune system for overall health) or the treated area.

f) Place a clear plastic sheet over the treated area followed by the heating pad. Set the heating pad on low and make adjustments if necessary.

g) Wrap the affected area with the white towel.

h) Castor Oil pack remains in place for 60 to 90 minutes and repeated daily - 03 to 07 days a week.

i) A plastic sheet may be placed on the bed if the castor pack is used while laying down or sleeping.

j) Castor Oil packs may be reused as long as the oil doesn't become rancid. You can place them in clear plastic bags and place them in your refrigerator.

For other areas when using Castor Oil for external use, use smaller flannel pieces. You may also use gauze pads and even band-aids.

If you have aching feet, saturate a pair of white socks in Castor Oil and wear some old shoes or slippers while walking around or when sleeping!

Again, many times Castor Oil packs are placed on the abdomen which gets the immune system to *"kick-in"* its healing power! For other treated areas, simply apply the Castor Oil pack directly over the treated area.

Can I take Castor Oil internally?
Yes, you can. I advise you to read any available materials on Castor Oil and I HIGHLY ADVISE you to seek advice from your physician.

What kind of Castor Oil should I get and where can I buy it?

Like Olive Oil, INSURE the Castor Oil you do by is:
a) Cold Pressed
b) Cold Processed
c) NO additives

Listed below are some Points Of Contact you should be aware of. See HomeHealth for a source to buy Castor Oil and reusable flannel cloth.

Association for Research
Enlightenment, Inc. (ARE)---------1-800-333-4499
                                   1-804-428-3588
                                   1-804-422-4631(fax)

Association for Research Enlightenment, Inc., (ARE) continues the work of a man named Edgar Cayce who founded the ARE in 1931. ARE is an international network of people and volunteers who are interested ancient civilizations, dream interpretation, ESP & psychic development, holistic healing, meditation, reincarnation, spiritual growth, the purpose of life, and much more. There are many benefits to ARE members such as: ARE Camp, ARE Conferences and Seminars, ARE books by mail, The New Millennium Journal, Venture Inward Magazine, and much more. They'll send you a catalog of their books. One of which is called The Oil That Heals (Castor Oil). Call Monday through Friday from 8:00 a.m. to 5:00 p.m., Eastern Standard Time, for your free information packet!

HomeHealth-Solutions For
Healthy Living------------------1-800-284-9123
HomeHealth, 3890 Park Central Blvd. North, Pompano Beach, FL 33064. HomeHealth is the *"Official Supplier of Edgar Cayce Products."* Home Health offers hundreds of healthy products like Castor Oil and Wool Flannel sheets. Other products are too numerous to mention. Their 40-page, all-color catalog is packed with super healthy products and even products for kittie and bowser! Call for your free all-color catalog today!

"Super Healthy Flaxseed Oil!"

You've already read about the amazing healthy possibilities of Shark Liver Oil, Olive Oil, and Omega-3 Fatty Acids. Now let's talk about one more healthy oil you have to know about - Flaxseed Oil!

In 1909, the average U.S. person consumed approximately 125 grams of fat per day. Today the average person in the U.S. consumes approximately 175 grams of fat, an increase of 40 percent or about 50 extra pounds per year and increasing!

Of the total increase in the consumption of fats and oils, shortening, margarine, refined salad oil and cooking oils account for fifty percent. This increase in fat over the years is undoubtedly linked to the increase in degenerative diseases.

In order to extend the shelf life of many products, essential fatty acids (good fat) have been purposely processed out of most foods. This is profitable for the manufacturer, but UNHEALTHY to the American consumer - YOU!

Approximately 80% of Americans are deficient in essential fatty acids. Flax seed has a high content of essential fatty acids.

Flax seed supplies the body with needed essential fatty acids and richer in Omega-3's than fish oil and packs more fiber ounce for ounce than oat bran!

Listed below are some observed benefits of flax seed:

- Seriously ill cancer patients were treated with flax seed oil and low-fat cottage cheese by Dr. Johanna Budwig. Over a period of approximately 90 days, tumors gradually receded. Symptoms of anemia, cancer, diabetes and liver dysfunction were completely alleviated!

- According to a study in Great Britain by Dr. Sinclair, a relative deficiency of the essential fatty acids plays an important part in the causes of arteriosclerosis, coronary thrombosis, diabetes mellitus, hypertension, multiple sclerosis and certain forms of malignant diseases!

- Dr. J.R. Vane shared the 1982 Nobel Prize for Medicine for his work proving how the metabolism of Omega-3 fatty acids helped prevent heart problems.

- A U.S. physician, Dr. Donald Rudin discovered that Omega-3 fatty acid deficiency is the basic cause of major mental illness, because fatty acids provide the substance upon which niacin and other B Vitamins act to form the prostaglandin-3 series tissue hormones which are special mission fatty acids that regulate neurocircuits through the whole body.

The Food and Drug Administration (FDA) has recently entered into a 03-year, $2 million contract with the National Cancer Institute (NCI) to research the effect of flax seed on various health concerns. The FDA will conduct experiments confirming flaxseed's role in fat and cholesterol metabolism, bone mineralization and the immune system. This research will make flaxseed one of the most intensively-studied nutrients used in any food product.

Flax seeds are a great source of healthy soluble and insoluble fiber as well as protein. Just 1/4 cup (50 grams) of flax seed provides 20 grams of fiber. Remember fiber is noted to ameliorate, heal, prevent:
- Colon cancer.
- Constipation.
- Diverticulosis.
- Hemorrhoids.
- Improves blood sugar metabolism.
- Lowers blood pressure.
- Lowers cholesterol.
- Protects against other cancers.
- Rectal cancer.
- Weight loss.
- Much more...

Follow the recommended dosage and instructions from the label and as per your doctor's instructions.

Here are two Points of Contact to get authentic Flaxseed Oil products.

Heintzman Farms-----------------1-888-333-5813
Heintzman Farms, Rural Route 2 Box 265, Onaka, SD 57466. Mr. Rick Heintzman owner of Heintzman Farms offers a kit that includes three 01-pound bags of Dakota Gold flax seed, an electric grinder and two home cholesterol test kits for only $70. If you want a free sample of flax seeds send a SASE! Heintzman Farms also offers 1-pound bags of flax seed or in bulk.

Nature's Distributors, Inc.,----1-800-624-7114
                                1-602-837-8420(fax)
Natures Distributors Inc., 16508 E. Laser Drive, Suite 104, Fountain Hills, AZ 85268. You have to look into this company. Not only do they have great products, but their advertisement reads *"place your first order with us, you will automatically receive the next 12 monthly issues of The Healthy Cell News."* I simply called them and asked for any literature about their products (to protect you from the bad companies). Nature's Distributors Inc., sent me The Healthy Cell News! One of the most informative health orientated subscriptions I have ever read! The Healthy Cell News is a full-size, 36-page, colorful, and extremely informative newspaper. Throughout the newspaper, you'll find and read about their healthy products. CALL them today! Call Monday through Friday from 8:00 a.m. to 4:00 p.m., Mountain Standard Time.

The previous Special Reports were taken from The
Gettysburg Program - What You Don't Know May Be Killing
You - Your Complete Guide To Vibrant Health.

Now let's carry-on with *"Super Fighting & Healing Oil
Of Oregano!"*

"Super Fighting & Healing Oil Of Oregano!"

Once you read this Special Report, I bet you're going to be so motivated to get this super healing wonder in your anxious hands, that you'll call the POC I'm going to give you within 10-seconds after you finish reading this very important Special Report.

This Special Report was taken directly from the 2005 Anytime Anywhere Survival Newsletter (2005 AASN) and is written in a Question and Answer format so you can better understand how powerful and important this healing wonder may be to you and your family member's benefit for the rest of your lives Anytime Anywhere! Are you ready? OK, let's get started with the history of healing oregano.

01) What is oregano and what is its healing history?
There are 60+ various species of oregano that come from the mint family, but very few oregano species have the super healing qualities we'll talk about in this Special Report. Oregano is commonly known as a seasoning herb, marjoram - (Origanum vulgare).

The antiseptic powers of oil of oregano are gigantic and make most other natural remedies and even synthetic drugs look weakly by comparison. Oil of oregano's wide and long resume of healings throughout history to the present day are very impressive (keep reading).

Without any assistance from other natural remedies or synthetic drugs, oregano kills fungus or blocks its growth. Oil of oregano also attacks and outright destroys antibiotic-resistant super-germs, bacteria, molds, parasites, viruses, yeast,...

In ancient times, the Greek Empire grew oregano along their hillsides. The Greeks used oregano for a variety of medicines which may explain why the Greeks were so powerful both mentally and physically.

Greek physicians used oregano to treat asthma, congestive heart failure, headaches, lung disorders, narcotic poisoning, open wounds, plant poisoning, seizures, venomous bites,... Approximately 3000 B.C., the Babylonians used oregano as a cure for lung and heart diseases. They also used oregano for treating wounds and venomous bites.

In the Middle Ages (476 AD to 1453 AD), Islamic physicians used oregano spices and oil of oregano as a germ killer. In the 9th century, a historian recorded that open markets in Baghdad, Iraq, sprinkled oregano on produce to keep it fresh. He recorded the vegetables went unspoiled for up to 02-weeks in the open air without any refrigeration.

Over thousands of years, oregano was eaten as food in the Mediterranean, Middle East, & Eastern Europe and each culture had their own oregano recipes. Some sprinkled oregano on their food while others added food to their oregano.

02) What types of healing oreganos are there?

There are oil of oregano, oregano juice, and crushed wild oregano. The crushed wild oregano, the entire herb in its natural state is processed by being sun-dried. Oregano juice is the water soluble extract of wild oregano and processed and extracted by steam distillation. Oil of oregano is also produced by steam distillation.

True healing oregano grows wild on rock or calcium-loaded soils. Oregano is loaded with minerals like boron, calcium, copper, iron, magnesium, manganese, phosphorus, potassium, zinc,... Ounce for ounce amazing super oregano has 16-times more calcium than milk. And its heavily loaded with zinc, ounce for ounce, more zinc than cheese, peanut butter, salmon, sardines,... Oregano also contains Vitamins like beta carotene, niacin, riboflavin (B complex), thiamine (B complex), Vitamin C, and Vitamin K. And oregano has anti-oxidant qualities, fighting free-radicals that cause disease, aging,... Oregano could be considered a super food.

03) What are the healing ingredients in oregano?

Oil of oregano contains a host of ingredients to carvacrol - its main ingredient. Carvacrol is a phenol which is a powerful antiseptic. It also contains another phenol called thymol. Together both phenols work synergistically, meaning the combination is more powerful together than alone.

Oil of oregano contains more than 50 compounds that possess antimicrobial functions with carvacrol and thymol being the main ingredients. Other ingredients include:

Alpha-humulene, Amyl Furan, Beta-Bisabolene, Beta-Caryophyllene, Camphene, Carene, Cineole, Cis-dihydrocarvone, Cis-sabinene Hydrate, Cymene, Decane, Germacrene D, Hexanal, Hexenal, Limonene, Linalool, Linalyl Acetate, Methyl Carvacrol, Myrcene, Nonanal, Nonane, Ocimene, Phellandrene, Pinene, Sabinene, Spathcoulane, Terpinen-4-ol, Terpinene, Terpinolene, Thymol, Trans-dihydrocarvone, Undecane,...

A study at Georgetown University Medical Center, Washington D.C., headed by Harry G. Preuss, M.D., tested the efficacy of oregano against Candida albicans (yeast infection) and found that oregano *"can act as a potent antifungal agent against Candida albicans."* Business Weekly magazine states *"Oregano could turn into the next wonder drug."*

04) Go back to the fungus part. Fungus is dangerous isn't it?
It surely is. Fungus lives off dead or dying tissue and it lives among live tissue outside and inside your body that causes all types of sickly maladies.

Listen to this, health-care in the United States runs more than a trillion dollars a year! Yet Americans are the most chronically sickliest people on Earth. More than 60% of all Americans are overweight. And Americans are the most fungally infested people on Earth and fungus is responsible for a many sickly maladies, some of which eventually leading to a costly sickly death.

Here's a good reason why Americans are the most fungally infested people on Earth. American love sugar, Americans are addicted to sugar. Just about every food, drink, and snack that is consumed by Americans has sugar in it. On the average, each American consumes a whopping 150-pounds of sugar each year! That's about 6 1/2-ounces of sugar each day! And that sugar is a food source for fungus, fungus that's inside you right now. No wonder you feel or are sick all the time.

And fungi is a survivor, it's difficult to kill. In nuclear bomb testing of the 1940s and 1950s, microbes were tested against radiation fallout. It turned out that Candida albicans, a fungus\yeast, survived the deadly fallout. Fungi is a survivor, difficult to kill, yet oil of oregano attacks and **kills fungi** easily, it's no contest.

And as I stated earlier, oil of oregano also attacks and outright destroys antibiotic-resistant super-germs, bacteria, molds, parasites, viruses, yeast,...

05) Why haven't I heard about super healing oregano before now?

The true healing oregano products haven't been around that long. They were introduced in the United States about 1996. At the same time there are federal laws prohibiting *"cure-all"* advertising. Plus, when folks do read the amazing super healing testimonials of oregano, most think it's too good to be true.

06) Are these super healing oregano products a cure-all?

It sure seems like they are but they're not, no one natural or man-made medicine is a cure-all. These super healing oregano products help your body to heal itself by going after the antibiotic-resistant super-germs, bacteria, fungus, molds, parasites, viruses, yeast,... inside and outside your body so your immune system can fight better to heal you.

With super healing oregano products, your immune system is no longer out-manned and out-gunned by antibiotic-resistant super-germs, bacteria, fungus molds, parasites, viruses, yeast,... invading your body.

07) What are some noted benefits of super healing oregano products?

Here's an exceptionally long list of what oregano kills (bad guys), as well as its benefits for ameliorating a wide variety of disorders. And this isn't a complete listing either.

Odds are YOU or someone close to you is troubled by one or more of the following health maladies and should take a closer look at super healing oil of oregano. OK, here's that list in alphabetical order:

Note: As I've always said *"Try the least intrusive method(s) first to remedy your health problem before going forward with conventional medicine of drugs and/or surgery."*

- Acne
- Alcoholic Neuritis
- Allergies
- Animal Bites
- Arthritis
- Asthma
- Athlete's Foot
- Back Pain
- Bad Breath
- Bed Sores
- Bladder Infections
- Boils
- Bromidrosis (body odor)
- Bronchitis
- Bruises
- Burns
- Bursitis
- Candidiasis
- Canker Sores
- Cellulitis
- Chicken Pox

- Cholera
- Colds
- Cold Sores
- Colitis
- Congestion
- Constipation
- Cough
- Crohn's Disease
- Croup
- Dandruff
- Dengue Fever
- Dental Cavities
- Dermatitis
- Diaper Rash
- Diarrhea
- Diphtheria
- Diverticulitis
- Ear Aches
- Ear Infections
- Ebola
- Eczema
- Emphysema
- Encephalitis (includes West Nile virus)
- Esophagitis
- Fatigue
- Fingernail Fungus
- Flactuence
- Flu

- Food Poisoning
- Frostbite
- Frostburn
- Gastritis
- Genital Herpes
- Giardiasis
- Gonorrhea
- Gout
- Gum Disease
- Hantavirus
- Headaches
- Hepatitis
- Hiatal Hernia
- Hives
- Impetigo (skin infection)
- Ingrown Toenail
- Insect Bites
- Irritable Bowel Syndrome
- Jock Itch
- Kidney Infection
- Kills Amebas
- Kills Antibiotic-Resistant Super-Germs
- Kills Bacteria
- Kills Camphylobacter
- Kills Clostridium
- Kills Cryptosporidium
- Kills Cyclospora
- Kills E. Coli

- Kills Enterobacter
- Kills Fleas
- Kills Flukes Cholera
- Kills Fungus
- Kills Germs
- Kills Giardia
- Kills Lice
- Kills Parasites
- Kills Salmonella
- Kills Shigella
- Kills Viruses
- Kills Worms
- Kills Yeast
- Laryngitis
- Leaky Gut Syndrome
- Leg Cramps
- Listeria
- Low Blood Pressure
- Lower Lung Conditions
- Lyme Disease
- Malaria
- Measles
- Mumps
- Nail Fungus
- Neuritis
- Open Wounds
- Oral Lesions
- Paronychia (nail infection)

- Peptic Ulcer
- Pneumatic Conditions
- Pneumonia
- Poison Ivy
- Poison Oak
- Poison Sumac
- Psoriasis
- Prostate Disorders
- Prostatis
- Pruritus (itchy skin)
- Radiation Injuries
- Rash
- Ring Worm
- Rosacea (face rash)
- Scabies
- Seborrhea
- Shingles
- Sinusitis
- Skin Cancer
- Sleeping Sickness
- Sore Throat
- Spider Bites
- Spinal Infection
- Splinters
- Sports Injuries
- Stomach Disorders
- Sunburn
- Tartar

- Tendinitis
- Thrush (mouth infection)
- Tick-borne Illness
- Tooth Abscess
- Toothache
- Tonsillitis
- Tuberculosis
- Upper Respiratory Tract Conditions
- Urinary Infection
- Varicose Veins
- Venomous Bites
- Vitiligo (skin pigment)
- Warts
- Wounds
- AND MORE...

08) How do I know how to use oregano for a particular malady?

First, so I won't get sued by some weasel money-hungry lawyer, I have to tell you that this Special Report like everything else in this IRISAP Survival Program is for *"informational use only."* Second, you must see your physician before you engage in any alternative supplement.

Odds are your doctor might say *"baaa hum bug"* and prescribe more drugs. However, YOU and YOU ALONE are the final approving authority for your precious health. Without your health, you got diddly squat - no matter how rich you are.

OK, now to answer your question. I'm way ahead of you, below is a GREAT book you have to get for valuable information on super healing oregano. This 203-page book will give you all the information you need to act upon for this super healing herb. Plus, when you send for FREE information from the POC below, they also give doses and instructions for their authentic oregano products.

09) Are there fake oregano products out there?

Yes, you bet there are. Not until 1996 were true medicinal oregano products available in the United States. Before this time and the present, fake oregano products appear on healthfood store shelves throughout the country. These fake oregano products have little or no medicinal qualities. Fake oregano products that carry the name but are products like marjoram oil, Spanish oregano, thyme oil,...

10) Where can I read more about super healing oregano?

Here is a book you have to get as soon as possible (beg borrow or go to your local library):

The Cure Is In The Cupboard-----by Dr. Cass Ingram (How To Use Oregano For Better Health). I used this book as one of my references for this Special Report.

11) Where can I get authentic oregano products?

Here's a POC recommended by Dr. Cass (author above) to get authentic oregano products and a lot more:

North American Herb & Spice-------1-800-243-5254
                                  1-847-473-4780

North American Herb & Spice, P.O. Box 4885, Buffalo Grove, IL 60089. North American Herb & Spice offers a wide variety of authentic oregano products as well as other healing products like: Oils of Basil, Bay Berry, Bay Leaf, Celery Seed, Cilantro-Plus, Cinnamon, Clove Buds, Cumin, Fennel, Ginger, Hpericum, Juniper, Lavender, Myrtle, Propolis, Rosemary, Sage, Wild Mint,... and Cardio Clenz, Flavin C, Intesti Clenz, Kidnee Clenz, Liva Clenz, Nuke Protect, Prosta Clenz, Scalp Clenz, Skin Clenz, ThyroKelp,... and they offer several healthy books to inform you of alternative therapies, medicines, home remedies,... I (author) highly recommend this POC. Call or write for FREE literature today.

"STOP Toothache Pain With This Super Oil!"

Folks, I want to make sure you get your money's worth, so here's another late entry. This is going to be very brief but extremely worthy of your attention when no dentist is available for a really bad toothache pain.

In late July of 2013, I was suffering from a non-stop toothache pain from hell. I swished and gargled with salt water which actually helped out a bit but the pain came back. I dental flossed repeatedly trying to remove any debris that may have been caught between the tooth and gum and I massaged the area practically non-stop trying to get more blood in the area. But the horrible toothache pain miserably occupied my life every second for about 02-days.

I gotta tell you, they could throw that water-boarding interrogation technique (Chinese Water Torture) out the window and give that prisoner a plain ol' fashion killer toothache from hell and that prisoner will soon start talking non-stop and beg for a dentist to relieve his awful pain.

As always, I conducted some *"intensive research"* to solve my aching problem. Finally, I think I found the healing answer to my toothache pain without spending several hundred dollars for an emergency dentist visit.

But to make sure I keyed on this healing oil and conducted more research or was it too occupy myself so to try to get my mind off the nagging toothache pain.

Well, I decided this oil was going to be my healer, my banishment for this cussing toothache. I got in my car and ended up driving at least 02-hours trying to this elusive oil. I tried GNC - they were out of it. I tried another GNC, they were closed. I tried Walgreen - what kind of oil did you say? I finally found a Mom & Pop health food store and they had it!!!

I purchased it and walked out the door and went to another store to buy some cotton balls and some Q-Tips. Returning to my car, I applied this Special Oil right in the parking lot.

OK, OK, what kind of oil are you talking about?

This special oil is called Clove Oil (*Eugenia caryophyllata*) {Ingredients: 100% pure clove oil}. The 01-fluid ounce (30 mL) dark bottle cost $6.99 plus taxes. Here's a step-by-step process of what I did to STOP my toothache in less than 02-minutes.

Step 01: Apply 03 or 04 drops of Clove Oil to a single Q-Tip.

Step 02: Massage the treated Q-Tip to the tooth or teeth for 15-seconds.

STEP 03: Massage the same treated Q-Tip to the surrounding gum area for 15-seconds.

Step 04: Go ahead and spit, cause Clove Oil has a strong scented taste to it.

STEP 05: Repeat Steps 01 thru 04. You'll find after the 1st treatment the toothache pain is already diminishing. At the end of the 2nd treatment, the toothache pain is completely gone – well this is what happened to me. And the toothache pain never returned.

Clove Oil goes after the bad guys (germicide, bactericide,…), so I think I had a bad infection and the Clove Oil went after it. Bottom line – it STOPPED my non-stop toothache pain within a couple minutes. I hope you can use this info in the future when no dentist is immediately available.

OK, now let's carry-on with *BONUS HEALING*!

BONUS HEALING!

Cold Water Cures: If there is one thing I hate more than 08-legged spiders, it's cold frigid water. I can still hold my own when it comes to cold weather to include being soaking wet with cold water (surface or submerged) but I just have a lot of *"Art Of Suffering"* bad miserable memories (military) when it comes to cold water. Anyway, did you know plain ol' cold water has some very beneficial healthy effects?

According to Gurudev Khar Khalsa, a noted Sat Nam Rasayan Healer and Kundalini Yoga Teacher from Los Angeles, California: *"Cold Water Massage Therapy is one of the healthiest and most inexpensive of therapies. Simply massage the body with almond oil before taking a shower. Shower in cold water until your body temperature rises and no longer feels cold, but toasty and warm. Make sure the bathroom is heated. Never get out of a cold shower into a cold room."*

And here's list maladies remedied by cold water and complimentary benefits of taking cold showers - Brrrrr:
- Acne
- Allergies
- Anxiety Attacks
- Asthma
- Awake
- Blood Cholesterol Lower
- Blood Circulation

- Blood Pressure Reduced
- Blood Sugar Lowered
- Body Feels Warmer
- Body Odor Eliminated
- Calming Effect
- Cleanses Circulatory System
- Clearer Mind
- Complexion
- Concentration Improvement
- Depression Eliminated
- Dry Skin
- Eliminates Poisons & Toxins
- Energy
- Feelings Of Euphoria
- Five Senses Improved
- Flushes Organs
- Focus Improvement
- Hair Improvement
- Headaches Eliminated
- Heart Problems
- Heightened Awareness
- Immune System Booster
- Learning Improvement
- Less\No Colds
- Less\No Flu
- Leg Bloating\Pain,...
- Libido Improvement
- Mental Faculties Improved
- Migraines Eliminated

- Mood Improvement
- Muscle Cramps
- Pain
- Panic Attacks
- Positive Thoughts
- Pulse Rate Lower
- Rashes
- Refreshed
- Skin Improvement
- Sinusitis
- Sleep Improvement
- Strengthens Nervous System
- Strengthens Mucous Membranes
- Stress Buster
- Sweating Reduced
- Utility Bill Reduced
- Zest For Life

I've told you before that the BLOOD RULES! It's apparent to me that cold showers get the blood moving thus the many benefits of plain ol' *Cold Water C*

Want More Proof? Then Read This:

Lake Baikal Fountain Of Youth: Lake Baikal is located in Siberia Russia, and it's the oldest and deepest freshwater lake (01-mile) in the world and complimented with 27 islands.

It holds more water than all 05 Great Lakes in the Unites States combined. And many Russians swear it may be a fountain of youth. Let's start with *Curative Mineral Baths*.

a) Curative Mineral Baths: Whether you know it or not your own body is made up of many minerals which are needed for a healthy vibrant life. And minerals can be absorbed via baths - hot baths that open your skin's pours. Over 800 people a week go to Goryachinsks, a hot springs resort on Baikal's eastern shore.

There, its patrons lazily soak in bathtubs filled with hot mineral waters straight from Baikal's underground hot springs. Many swear that Baikal's hot springs cured their sickly maladies.

b) Rejuvenating Waters: Lake Baikal's Siberian waters are killer cold. Its waters invite hypothermia with open arms. But on the other side of the coin, its waters may be the Fountain Of Youth! Yuri and Sasha take part in the traditional Russian *banya*.

Banya is bathing in a hot steam bath followed by a dip through a ice hole into super cold water. As Yuri brags *"Baikal makes you feel young again, like baby!"* Sasha adds *"Like you have milk in blood!"* (Taken from National Geographic - June 1992)

Want More Proof?   Then Read This:

Back Pain Remedy: One of the crew members - Bratton (1805 - Lewis & Clark Expedition), was suffering from severe back pain. His back pain was so severe he had trouble just sitting up. So, Captain Clark used an Indian application that actually healed Bratton's back problem. A 04-foot deep pit was dug out. A fire built inside the pit with rocks added to retain heat. Horsemint tea was added with Bratton sitting in the pit enveloped in the steam.

After several minutes in this sweat bath, Bratton was carried away and submerged in cold water. After a quick cold dip, he was returned to the home-made wet sauna bath. The repeated hot-cold, hot-cold treatment was repeated several times. After several applications, Bratton was wrapped in a blanket. His back pain improved the next day and he soon recovered completely.

1st Note: Horsemint includes several course aromatic plants like Mentha Longifolia.

2nd Note: This is a perfect example of an alternative medicine called Hydrotherapy. Here's a quote from the Gettysburg Program: ****"*Hydrotherapy is the use of water, ice, steam and hot and cold temperatures to maintain and **restore health**.*

59

Treatments include full body immersion, steam baths, saunas, sitz baths, colonic irrigation and the application of hot and\or cold compresses. Hydrotherapy is effective for treating a wide range of conditions and can easily be used in the home as part of a self-care program."

Want More Proof? Then Read This:

Here's a true story how cold water can preserve the body and defy the sure-grip of DEATH!

Cold Water Diving Reflex - They're Still Alive: Folks, one of the most unforgiving environments are frigid cold weather environments. Worse yet are killer cold water environments. The human body is not designed to hold-up in cold weather environments for any length of time or even short periods. Once the core temperature drops below 98.6 degrees Fahrenheit - problems arise and get worse real quick the lower the body temperature drops. Simple shivering is a sign of hypothermia.

As I said, killer cold water environments are the worst. But there may be a way to bring back the dead, it's called *Cold Water Diving Reflex*. Let me go back in time and tell you a true story so you can better understand *Cold Water Diving Reflex*.

Several years ago, during the cold winter months in Fargo, North Dakota, an 11-year old boy with his sled was having fun like any other boy with his sled. The boy and his sled were over frozen water when he fell through the ice. Fargo Rescue and other nearby departments were soon dispatched to the scene. Rescue workers deployed their boats into the water, breaking the ice and probing for the boy's body with grappling poles.

As more and more minutes went by, one would think that there was no hope for the young boy. But the rescue workers knew something most people are unaware of - it's called *Cold Water Diving Reflex*.

Cold Water Diving Reflex not only retards the metabolism but puts the body's main organs in suspended animation to hold-off death! The multiple rescue workers were betting that if they found the boy real soon, *Cold Water Diving Reflex* would help them save the boy.

After 45 minutes underwater, the boy was finally hooked - they found him. He was brought into the boat where they brought him to shore. His body temperature was only 77-degrees - he was DEAD DEAD! Immediate CPR was applied to the boy on the way to the hospital.

The paramedics revived the boy! At the hospital, the young boy made a full recovery! He was under the frigid water for 45-minutes and survived! He survived because of *Cold Water Diving Reflex*!

Now I'm not sure if *Cold Water Diving Reflex* applies only to children only or if it also apples to adults. This subject RFIR. If you know any firemen, paramedics, doctors,... ask them and let me know what they say.

Now you understand why I keep telling you *"NEVER give-up, there's always a solution."*

Before I end this subject, I want to give you some data on hypothermia survival and ice support thickness.

Hypothermia Water Survival Table

Water Temp	Exhaustion & Unconscious Time	Max Survival Time
32.5 F	15-min	15-45 min
32.5-40F	15-30min	30-90 min
40-50F	30-60min	01-03 hrs
50-60F	01-02hrs	01-06 hrs
60-70F	02-07hrs	02-40 hrs
70-80F	03-12hrs	03 hours+

NOTE: Other considerations are the survivor's swimming abilities, predators, prior cold injuries, other injuries, available flotation equipment or floating debris, weather conditions, survivor's attitude, and other survivors present and their status (above considerations).

Ice Support Measurements!

You & Equipment Weigh ??? -	Ice Should Be
One survivor - no equipment	02-inches thick
Group of Survivors in a file	03-inches thick
Car or snowmobile (02 tons)	07.5-inches thick
Light truck (02.5 tons)	08-inches thick
Medium truck (03.5 tons)	10-inches thick
Heavy truck (09 tons)	12-inches thick
10 tons of weight	15-inches thick
25 tons of weight	20-inches thick

NOTE: Before you venture on frozen ice (lakes, ponds...), insure you see the local Forest Ranger for best and up-to-date safe ice-thickness measurements. If you're in a survival environment, walk around the frozen water obstacle.

More Survival Kindle E-Books And Survival Paperback Books For YOU!

Joseph A. Laydon Jr. (MSG Ret. Army) is the author and owner of Intensive Research Information Services And Products (IRISAP). Joseph has been writing *"self-reliance"* orientated data since 1991 and since July 2012 has been re-publishing his works via Kindle E-Books and Kindle Paperback Books. He has self-published more than **100+ Survival Books** (Kindle E-Books and Kinde Paperback Books). Below is a list of all his Survival Books and you can see these books by simply going to the website listed below for detailed descriptions and videos. See *"About The Author."*

- **Kindle E-Books:**-----------www.survivalexpertblog.com/52-survival-books/

- **Kindle Paperback:**-------www.survivalexpertblog.com/52-survival-books/

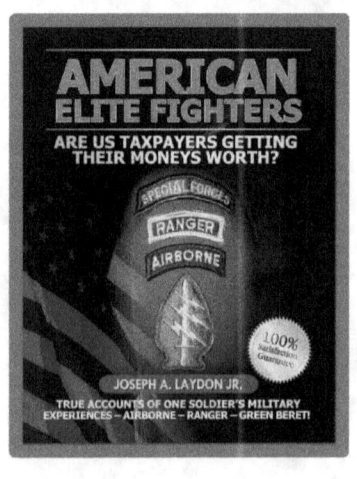
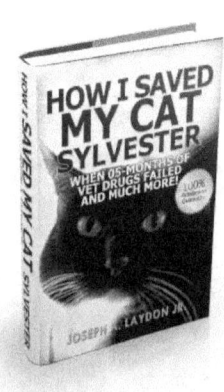
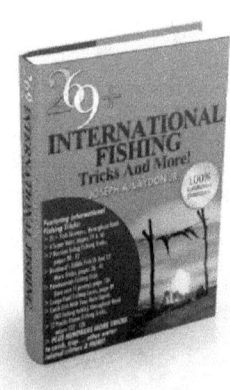

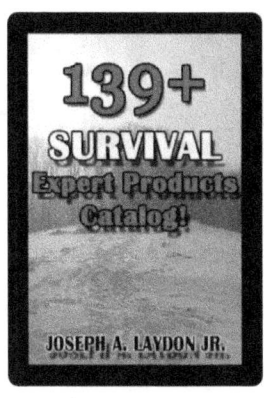

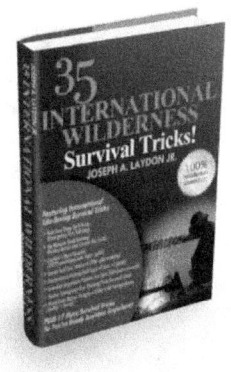

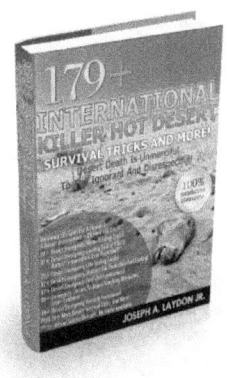

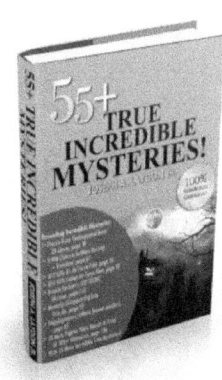

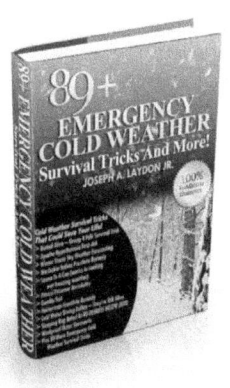

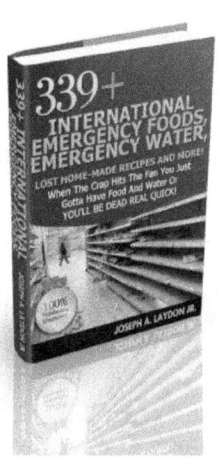

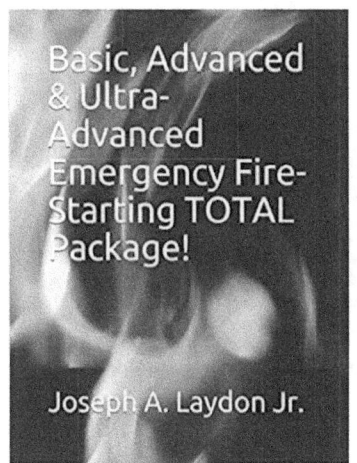

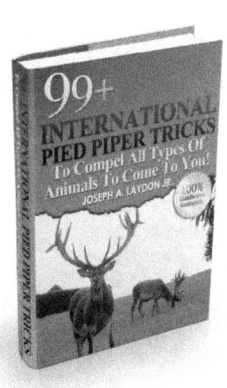

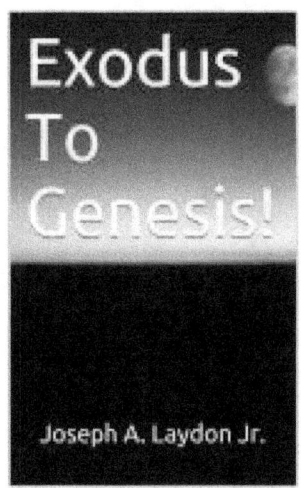

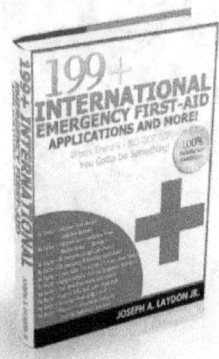

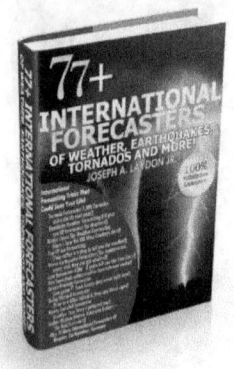

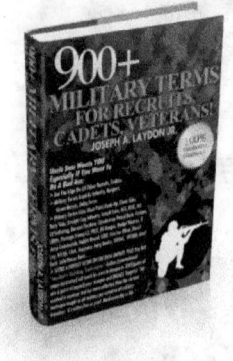

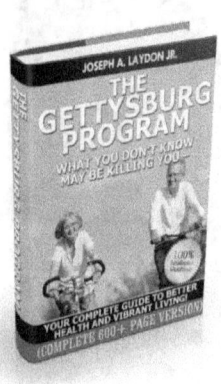

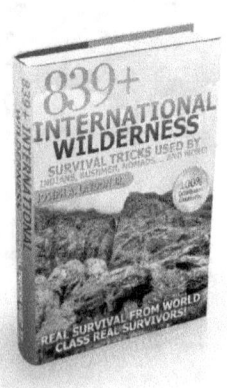

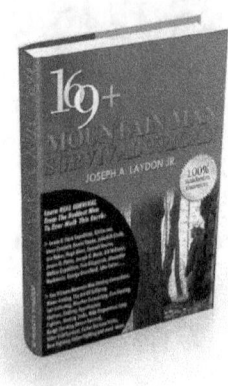

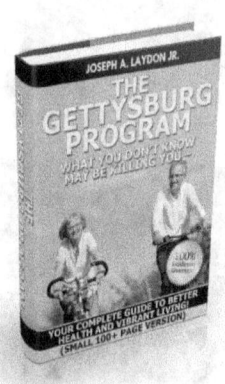

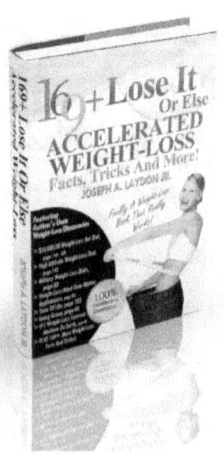

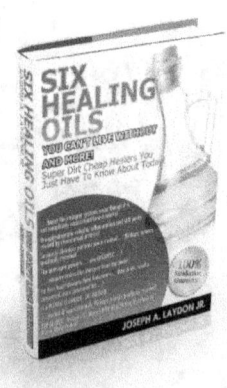

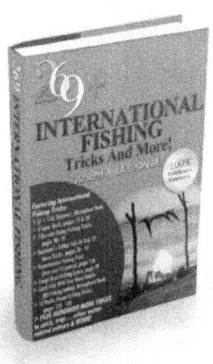

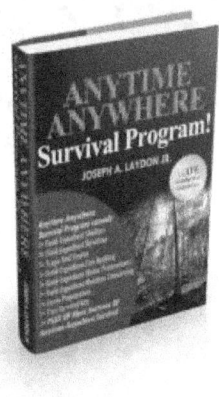

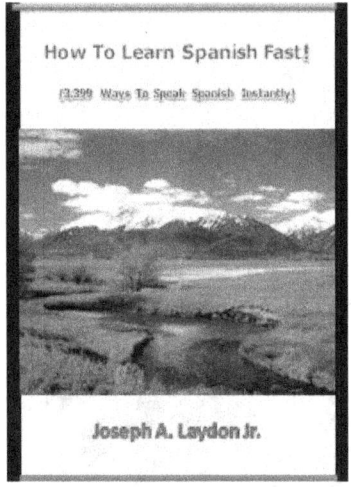

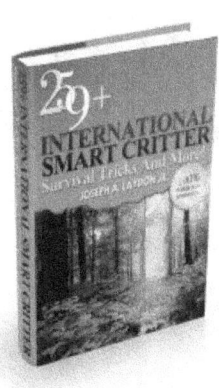

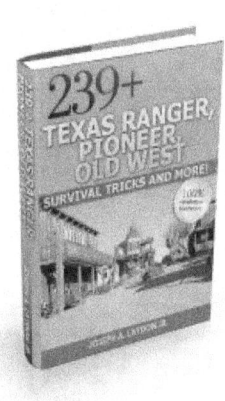

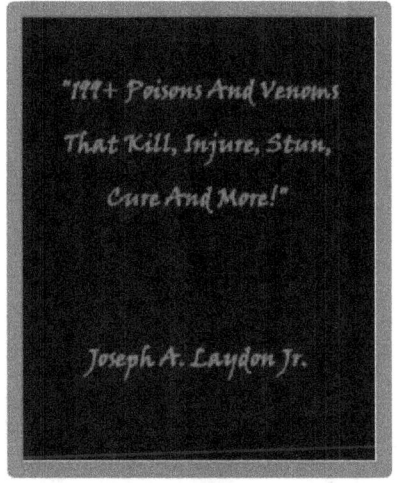

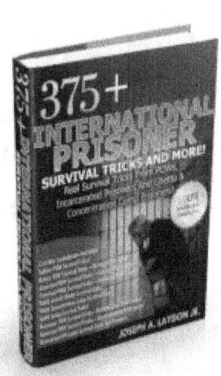

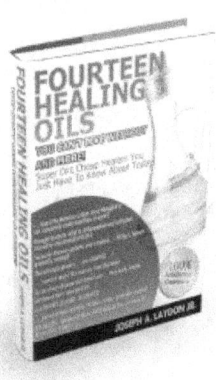

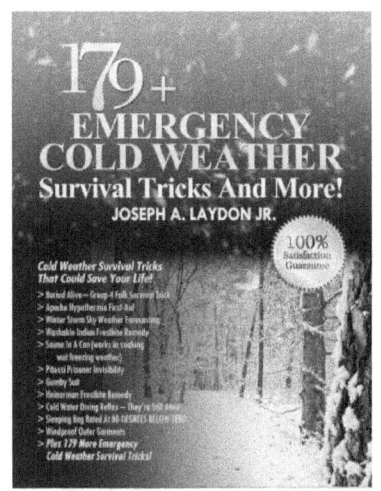

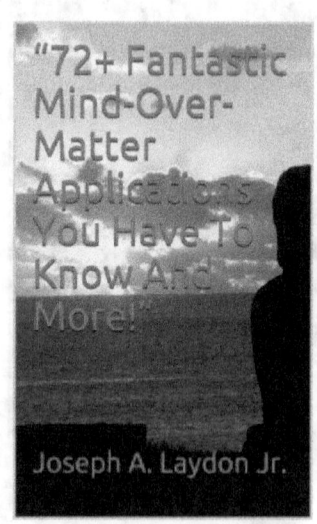

"72+ Fantastic Mind-Over-Matter Applications You Have To Know And More!"

Joseph A. Laydon Jr.

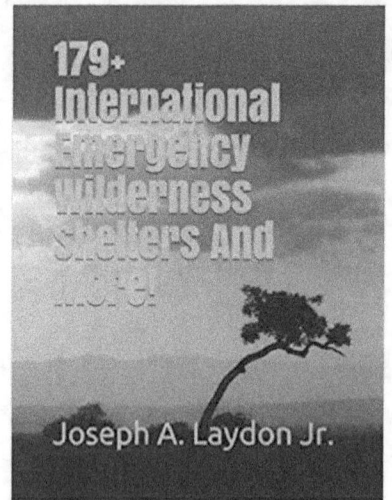

179+ International Emergency Wilderness Shelters And More!

Joseph A. Laydon Jr.

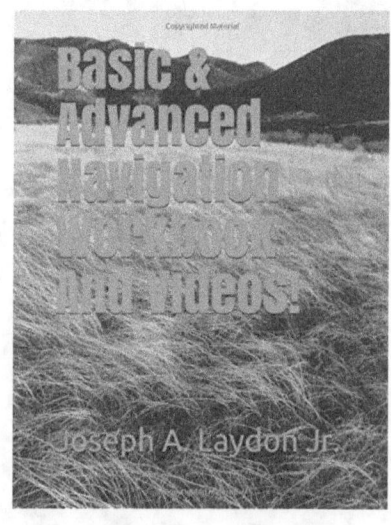

Basic & Advanced Navigation Workbook and Videos!

Joseph A. Laydon Jr.

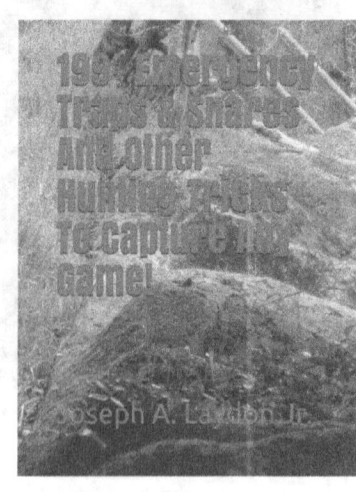

198+ Emergency Traps & Snares And Other Hunting Tricks To Capture Your Game!

Joseph A. Laydon Jr.

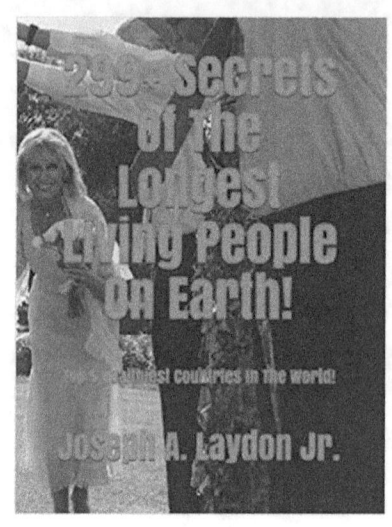

299+ Secrets Of The Longest Living People On Earth!

Top 5 Healthiest Countries In The World!

Joseph A. Laydon Jr.

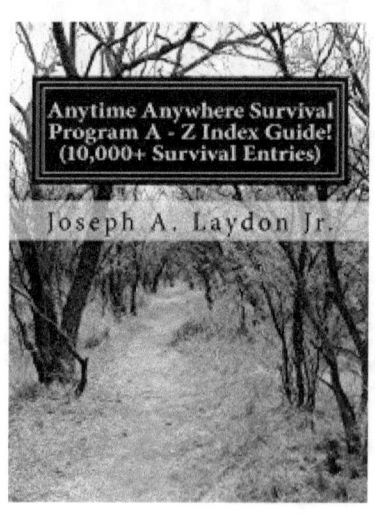

Anytime Anywhere Survival Program A - Z Index Guide! (10,000+ Survival Entries)

Joseph A. Laydon Jr.

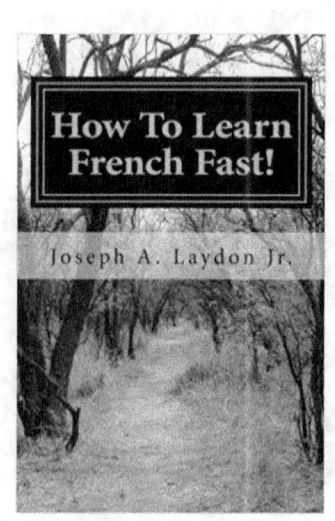

How To Learn French Fast!

Joseph A. Laydon Jr.

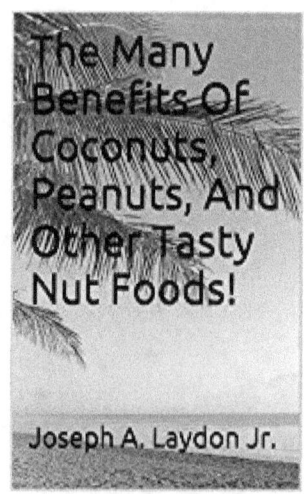

The Many Benefits Of Coconuts, Peanuts, And Other Tasty Nut Foods!

Joseph A. Laydon Jr.

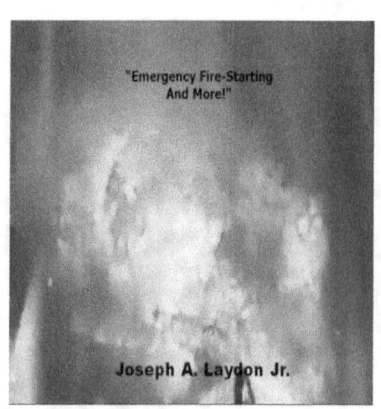

"Emergency Fire-Starting And More!"

Joseph A. Laydon Jr.

99+ International Diabetes Preventers, Fighters, Killers And More!

Joseph A. Laydon Jr.

99+ International Heart Attack Preventers, Fighters, Killers And More!

Joseph A. Laydon Jr.

99+ International Cancer Preventers, Cancer Fighters, Cancer Killers And More!

Joseph A. Laydon Jr.

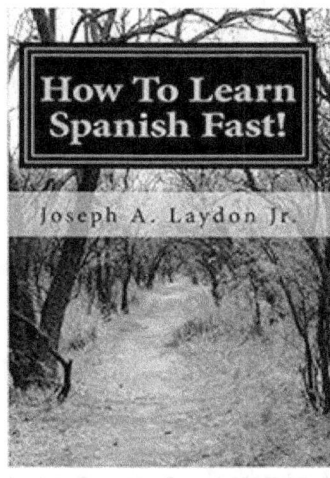

How To Learn Spanish Fast!

Joseph A. Laydon Jr

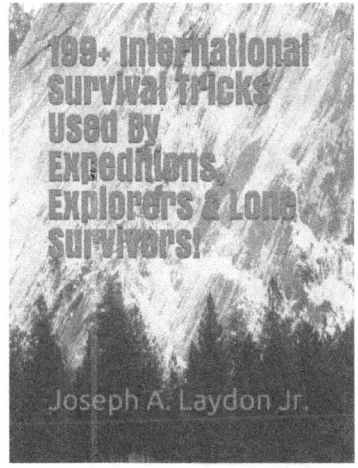

199+ International Survival Tricks Used By Expeditions, Explorers & Lone Survivors!

Joseph A. Laydon Jr.

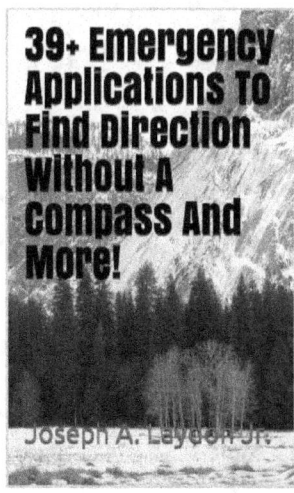

39+ Emergency Applications To Find Direction Without A Compass And More!

Joseph A. Laydon Jr.

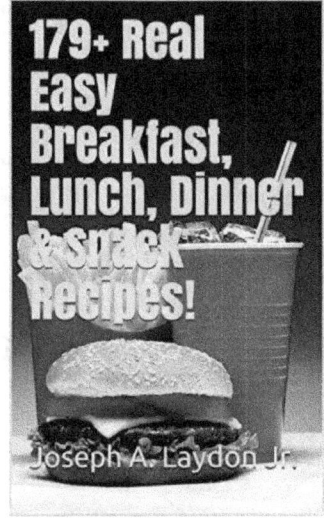

179+ Real Easy Breakfast, Lunch, Dinner & Snack Recipes!

Joseph A. Laydon Jr.

99+ Healings And Cures You Have To Know And More!

Joseph A. Laydon Jr.

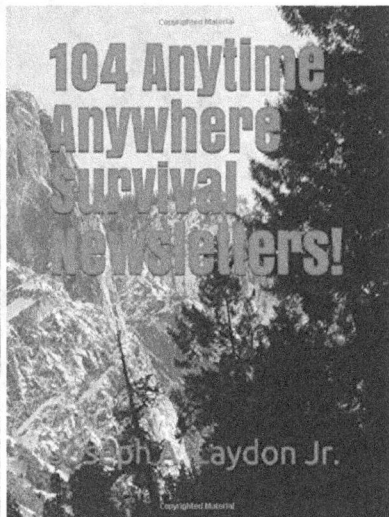

104 Anytime Anywhere Survival Newsletters!

Joseph A. Laydon Jr.

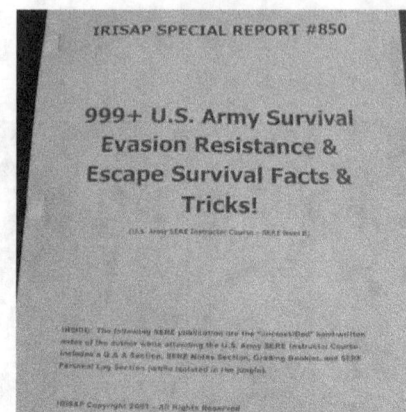

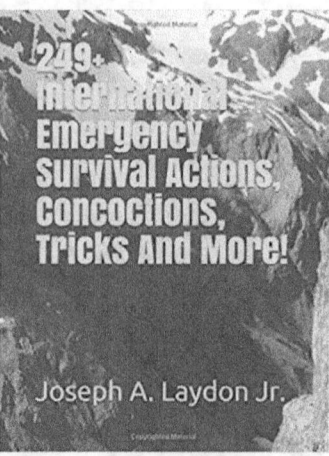

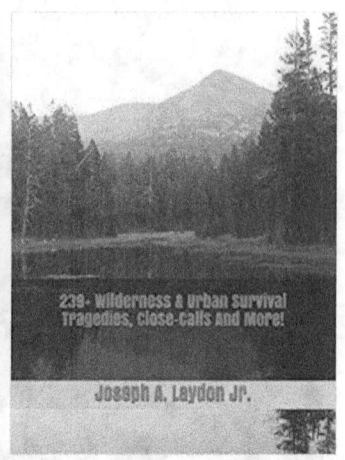

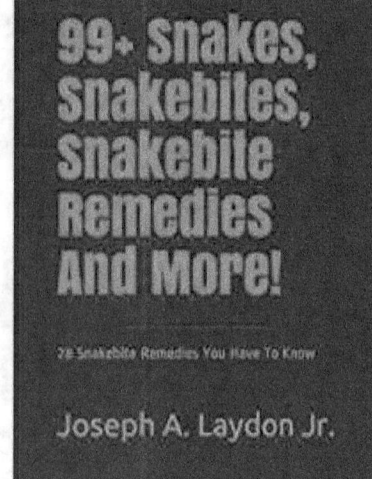

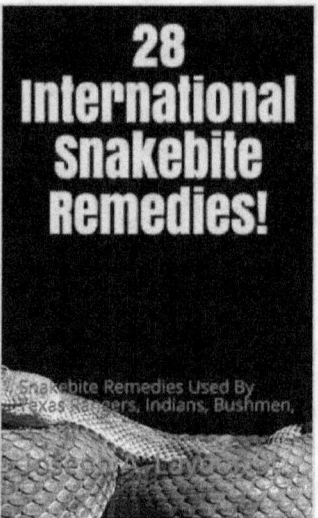

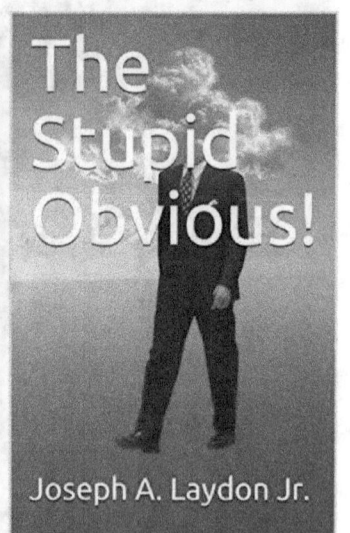

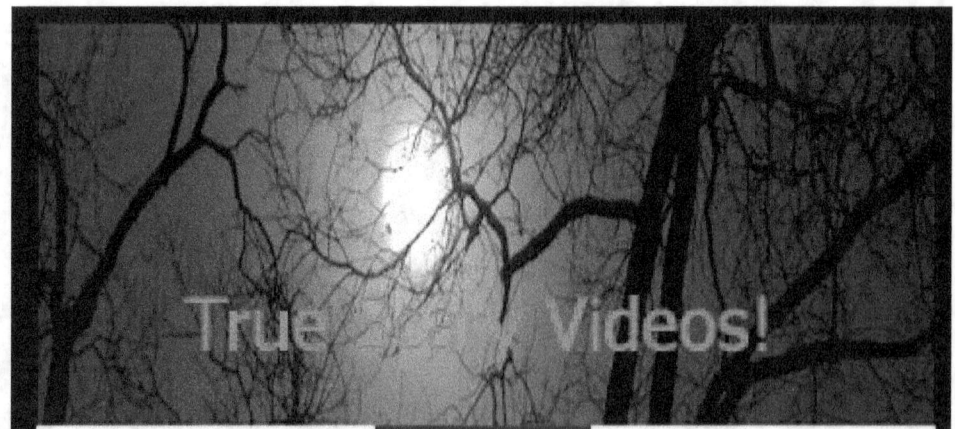

www.truescaryvideos.com

About The Author

Joseph A. Laydon Jr. (MSG (E-8) Retired United States Army - 18Z5V) is the author and owner of *Intensive Research Information Services And Products (IRISAP)*. Joseph is a
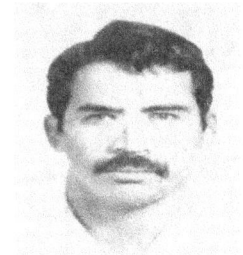 well-qualified instructor in international wilderness survival and the other 03 Survivals he teaches (Health Survival, Crime Survival and Money Survival). He is a 20-year U.S. Army veteran (Master Sergeant E-8 - 18Z5V) associated with all Special Operations units in the U.S. military, as well as Special Ops units in the Mid-East and Central & South America.

He's a qualified SERE Instructor (Survival Evasion Resistance & Escape) and has **taught wilderness survival** at the college level for 03 years. He's a qualified instructor in basic & advanced pistol marksmanship, basic & advanced rifle marksmanship, CQB (Close Quarter Battle), basic & advanced cross-country navigation, basic mountaineering techniques, and self-defense. Since 1994, he's published many self-improvement Survival Programs, Survival Videos, SPECIAL Reports, Intelligence Reports, monthly Newsletters, **100+ Survival Books** (Kindle E-Books & Kindle Paperback Books) and more in the works.

He's an inventor, he *"sideways engineers"* new survival tricks that can SAVE YOUR LIFE! An example: On 17 August 2000 - 1417 hours, at Scott Lake, Scott AFB, IL, Joseph made international history! He is the 1st in the world to replicate the mysterious fires of Africa using a single drop of water! On 05 January 2001, he discovered how to start a life-saving fire in just 02-seconds using a beam of light from a flashlight in pitch black *"blind man"* darkness! On 06 April 2005 - 1810 hours, he invented delicious & tasty Solid Fuel Rolls and several Trail-Mix Cookies that are used as emergency foods and used as long-burning emergency fire-starting kindling.

And recently - **50+ MORE TOP SECRET INVENTIONS** of advanced & **ultra-advanced fire-starting** like starting EMERGENCY FIRE-STARTING using personal care products and first-aid products you already use like:
- Shampoo
- Toothpastes
- Mouthwashes
- Breath Drops & Breath Sprays
- Salves
- Ointments
- Over-The-Counter Medicines
- Drink Enhancement Products
- Other ingredients like your spit (saliva), your urination,...

See **www.survivalexpertblog.com/save-my-life-survival-program**

He also teaches Advanced Navigation (*Basic & Advanced Navigation Workbook And Videos* [includes Workbook, Videos, maps, protractors,…]) so you're ready Anytime Anywhere! Only from IRISAP and only for privileged IRISAP subscribers - YOU! See *Basic & Advanced Navigation Workbook And Videos at* the end of this Survival Book.

Below is a sample of his military achievements & qualifications (**not in chronological order**) which reflect his unique & superior ability to teach basic, advanced & ultra-advanced survival applications, techniques and "tricks" that could help you AVOID serious killer survival threats as well as SAVE YOUR LIFE when you get in life or death situations. His trade secrets, Programs, and Videos are only offered to IRISAP subscribers-YOU!

- U.S. Army Airborne School
- U.S. Army Special Forces Qualification Course - SFQC (Green Beret)
- U.S. Army Master Parachutist Wings
- Uruguayan Parachutist Wings
- British Parachutist Wings
- Kingdom of Jordan Parachutist Wings
- Expert Infantry Badge - EIB
- 82nd Airborne Division Recondo Course
- Adverse Weather Aerial Delivery System Tests - AWADS (01 of 386 volunteer paratroopers)
- U.S. Army Special Forces Weapons Course (U.S. & foreign pistols, submachineguns, assault rifles, rifles, machineguns, mortars, anti-tank weapons, anti-aircraft weapons,…)
- Weapons Armorer Course
- Indirect Fire Course (60mm, 81mm, & 4.2 inch *"four deuce"* mortars)
- Jumpmaster Course
- Basic French Language Course
- Combat Infantry Badge - CIB
- U.S. Army Ranger Course
- Advanced Navigation Course
- Special Forces Sniper Course (02)
- Survival Evasion Resistance and Escape Instructor Course (SERE Level B)
- Wilderness Survival Instructor (College level - 03 years / 1991 - 1994)
- Rappell Master
- Fast Rope Master
- International Sniper Instructor
- International Close Quarter Battle (CQB) Instructor
- Participated In Multiple Combat Actions
- Special Forces Operations And Intelligence Course (O&I)
- Good Conduct Medal (06)
- Army Commendation Medal
- Army Achievement Medal (02)
- Meritorious Service Medal (02)
- Armed Forces Expeditionary Medal
- Letters Of Commendation (13)
- Letters Of Appreciation (08)

- Infantry Advanced NCO Course (11B)**
- Infantry Officer Basic Course **
- Military Intelligence Officer Basic Course **
- Held **SECRET** and **TOP SECRET** Clearances for 20+ years

** = These are military home study correspondence courses which took years to complete. This demonstrates Mr. Laydon's dedication to duty and desire to go beyond the training standards set by the U.S. Army Special Forces. You won't find too many soldiers completing years of military home study courses on their own time off. This reflects the author's many superior Survival Products like this Survival Product.

Featured on FOX-2 (24 August 2000). Joseph now resides in Illinois. He offers products concerning Wilderness Survival, Health Survival, Crime Survival and Money Survival so to greatly enhance the lives of all IRISAP subscribers - YOU! Any questions, write to Joseph today.

Sincerely,
Joseph A. Laydon Jr. (IRISAP)
P.O. Box 48
Cutler, IL 62238-0048

You And Yours Have A Safe One
Anytime Anywhere,

Joseph A. Laydon Jr.

E-Mail: wwwsurvivalexpert@yahoo.com

E-Mail: josephlaydonjr@gmail.com

WEBSITES

- Main Website--------------------www.survivalexpertblog.com
- 50+ Survival Paperback Books-----www.survivalexpertblog.com/52-survival-books/
- 50+ Survival Kindle E-Books------www.survivalexpertblog.com/52-survival-books/
- Anytime Anywhere Survival--------www.anytimeanywheresurvival.com
- Weight-Loss----------------------www.loseitorelseweightloss.com
- True Scary Videos----------------www.truescaryvideos.com
- Exodus To Genesis (Fiction Book)-www.exodustogenesis.com
- Survival Expert------------------www.survivalexpert.com
- Be On Survivor-------------------www.beonsurvivor.com
- Survival Expert Books------------www.survivalexpertbooks.com
- Survival Expert E-Books----------www.survivalexpertebooks.com
- Newsletters---------------------www.survivalnewsletters.com
- **NEW** - 'Survival Expert Blog'--https://www.survivalexpertblog.com

Take Notes

Take Notes

Take Notes

Take Notes

Take Notes

Take Notes

Take Notes

Take Notes

"Fourteen Healing Oils You Can't Live Without And More!"

THANK YOU, THANK YOU, THANK YOU for getting this Health Survival Book. I want to let you know there is a <u>BIGGER VERSION</u> of this Book (145-pages).

It's titled *"Fourteen Healing Oils You Can't Live Without And More!"* and gives you more oils you have to know about to benefit you today and decades into the future. PLUS, I give other very beneficial health information that is very worthy of your attention.

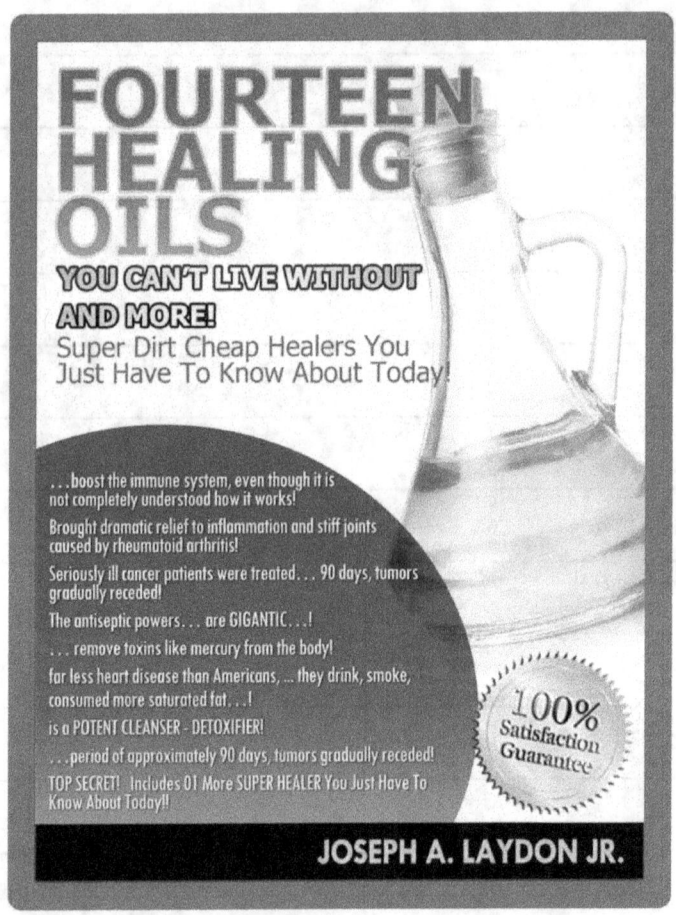

www.survivalexpertblog.com/52-survival-books

(Paperback Books)

www.survivalexpertblog.com/52-survival-books

(Kindle E-Books)

"More Heathy Books Worthy Of Your Attention!"

THANK YOU, THANK YOU, THANK YOU for getting this Health Survival Book. I want to let you know there are other Healthy Books that are worthy of your attention. I want to tell you, I am not a doctor nor am I qualified in any health profession. My job is I do research – "Intensive Research.". Here are some of my other 'health related' books that are worthy of your attention.

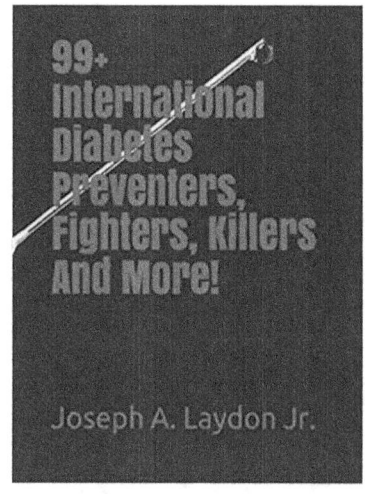 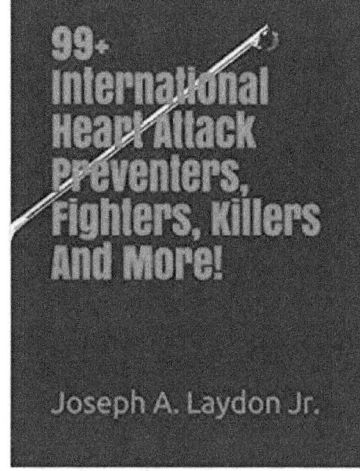 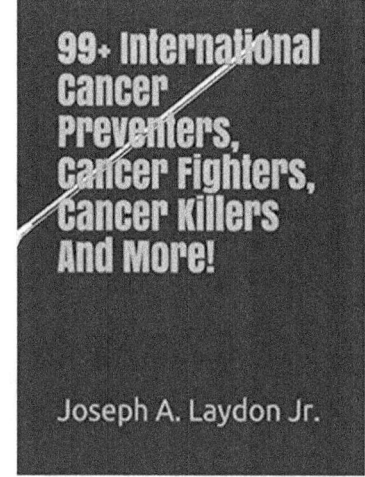

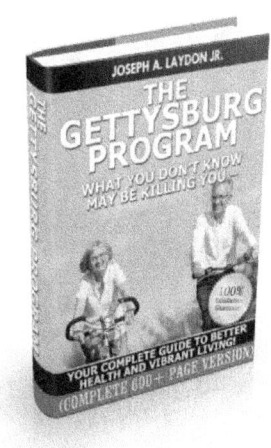 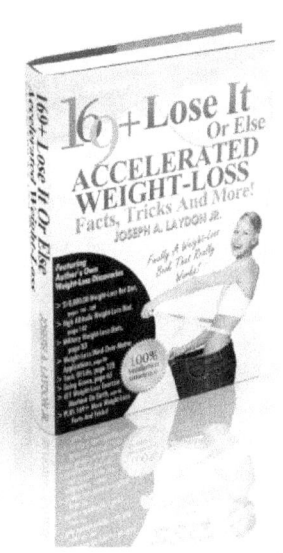 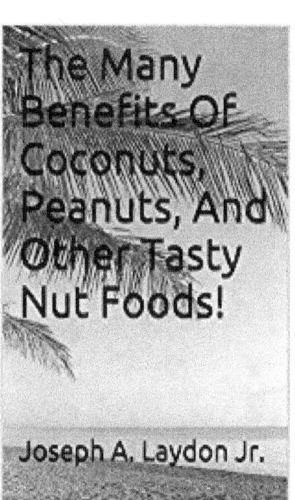

www.ingramcontent.com/pod-product-compliance
Lightning Source LLC
Chambersburg PA
CBHW081235280526
45787CB00006B/2665